THE BEST KETO FRIENDLY, SOUTH BEACH DIET

VERY EASY RECIPES TO BUSY PEOPLE EASY KETO DINNERS

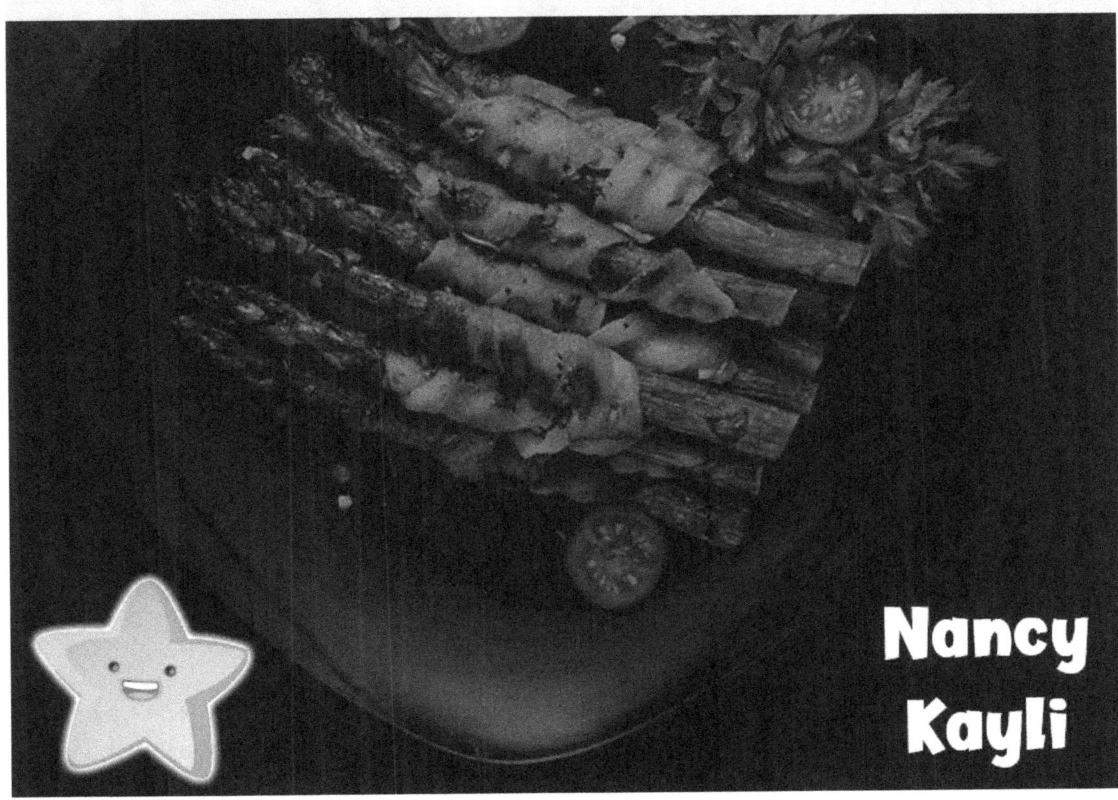

Nancy Kayli

The Best Keto Friendly, South Beach Diet

Very Easy Recipes To Busy People, Easy Keto Dinners

INTRODUCTION

Ketosis is a metabolic state in which your body uses fat and ketones rather than glucose (sugar) as its main fuel source.

Glucose is stored in your liver and released as needed for energy. However, after carb intake has been extremely low for one to two days, these glucose stores become depleted.

Your liver can make some glucose from amino acids in the protein you eat via a process known as gluconeogenesis, but

not nearly enough to meet the needs of

your brain, which requires a constant

fuel supply.

In ketosis, your body produces ketones

at an accelerated rate. Ketones, or

ketone bodies, are made by your liver

from fat that you eat and your own body

fat.

The three ketone bodies are beta-hydroxybutyrate (BHB), acetoacetate, and acetone (although acetone is technically a breakdown product of acetoacetate).

Even when on a higher-carb diet, your liver actually produces ketones on a regular basis mainly overnight while you sleep – but usually only in tiny amounts. However, when glucose and insulin levels decrease on a carb-restricted diet, the liver ramps up its production of ketones in order to provide energy for your brain.

<u>NUTRITIONAL DISCLAIMER</u>

Please note that I am not a medical or nutritional professional. I am simply recounting and sharing my own experiences on this book. Nothing expressed here should be taken as medical advice and you should consult with your doctor before starting any diet or exercise program.

I provide nutritional information for my recipes simply as a courtesy to my readers.

It is calculated using software and I remove erythritol from the final carb count and net carb count, as it does not affect my own blood glucose levels. I do my best to be as accurate as possible but you should independently calculate nutritional information on your own before relying on them. I expressly disclaim any and all liability of any kind with respect to any act or omission wholly or in part in reliance on anything contained in this website.

CHEESEBURGER SPAGHETTI SQUASH CASSEROLE

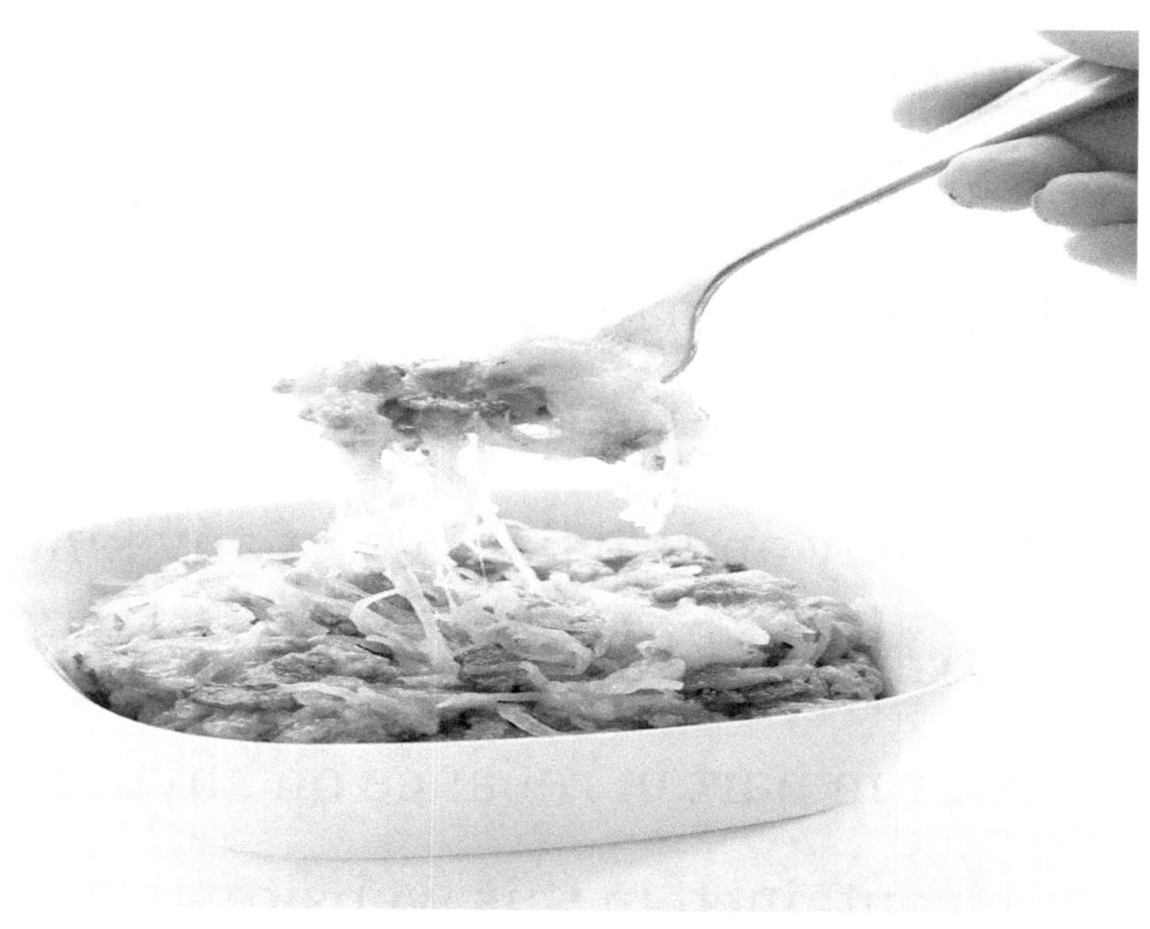

An easy Keto Cheeseburger Casserole recipe with spaghetti squash. This simple skillet casserole is the whole meal in one pan and it's delicious and filling. Topped with bacon for extra flavour and family appeal!

Prep Time: 10 mins

Cook Time: 1 hr 15 mins

Total Time: 1 hr 25 mins

Servings: 6 servings

Calories: 431 kcal

Ingredients

- 1 medium spaghetti squash

- 4 slices bacon, chopped

- 1 lb ground beef

- 2 cloves garlic, minced

- 1/2 tsp salt

- 1/2 tsp pepper

- 2 tbsp sugar free ketchup

- 2 tsp Worcestershire sauce

- 6 ounces shredded Cheddar (about 1 1/2 cups)

Instructions

1. Preheat the oven to 400F and line a baking sheet with parchment paper. Cut the squash in half crosswise and scoop out the seeds. Set the squash cut-side down and bake until the squash is soft enough to be squeezed, about 40 minutes.

2. Meanwhile, cook the bacon in a large skillet over medium heat until crisp. Remove to a paper towel lined plate.

In the same skillet, cook the ground beef, breaking up any clumps with the back of a wooden spoon.

3. When the beef is almost cooked through, about 7 minutes, add the garlic, salt, and pepper. Cook until no longer pink, another 2 or 3 minutes.

4. Stir in the ketchup and Worcestershire sauce. Scoop the flesh out of the squash and stir in until well mixed into the ground beef. Spread out evenly over the bottom of the skillet

5. Sprinkle with the shredded cheddar cheese and cover the skillet. Reduce the heat to low and let the cheese melt, about 5 minutes. Sprinkle the bacon overtop and serve.

Nutrition Facts

Amount Per Serving (1 serving = about 1 cup)

Calories 431Calories from Fat 259

% Daily Value*

Total Fat 28.8g44%

Total Carbohydrates 6.5g2%

Dietary Fiber 1.6g6%

Protein 30.5g61%

- Percent Daily Values are based on a 2000 calorie diet.

EASY TACO PIE

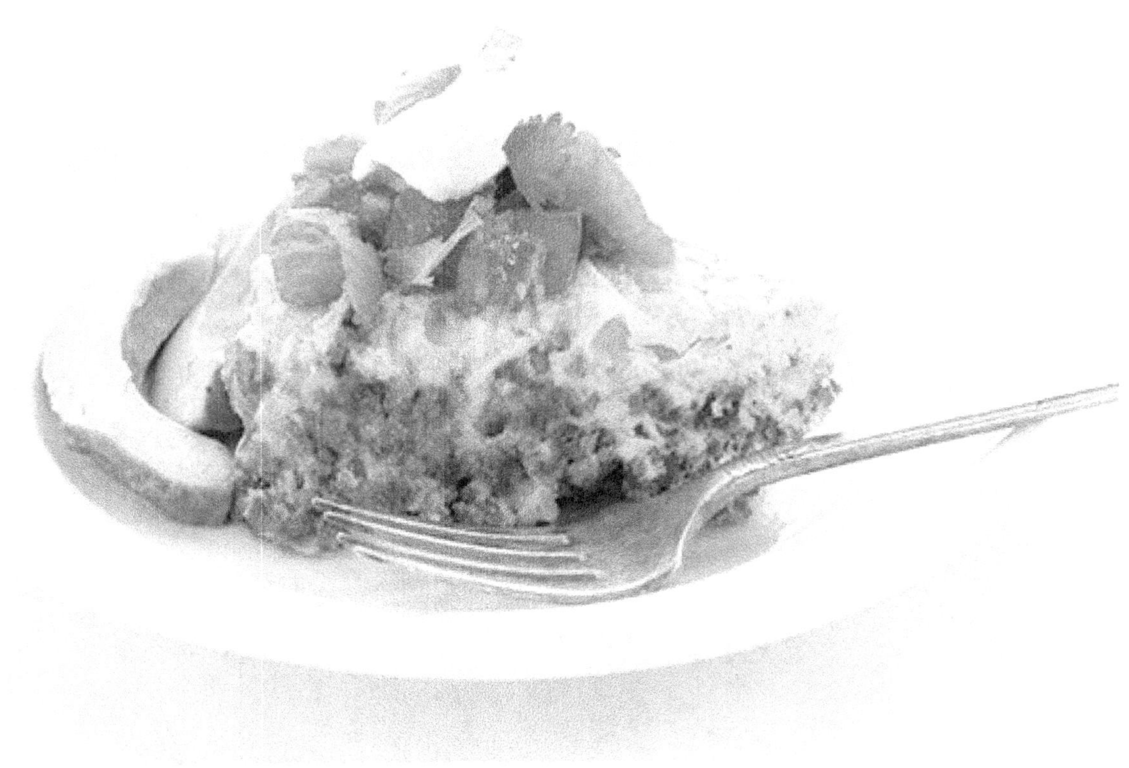

Prep Time: 15 mins

Cook Time: 30 mins

Total Time: 45 mins

This low carb taco pie is ridiculously easy to make and incredibly delicious - a perfect weeknight dinner. Use your favourite taco seasoning and adjust the heat to your liking. The whole family loves this easy keto dinner recipe.

Servings: 8 servings

Calories: 370 kcal

Ingredients

- 1 lb ground beef

- 3 tbsp taco seasoning or one packet taco seasoning

- 6 large eggs

- 1 cup heavy cream

- 2 cloves garlic minced

- 1/2 tsp salt

- 1/4 tsp pepper

- 1 cup shredded Cheddar cheese I used Cabot Chipotle Cheddar for an extra kick!

Instructions

1. Preheat oven to 350F and grease a glass or ceramic 9-inch pie pan.

2. Brown ground beef in a large skillet over medium heat until no longer pink, about 7 minutes, breaking up clumps with the back of a wooden spoon.

3. Add taco seasoning and stir until combined, then reduce heat to medium low and cook a few minutes longer until sauce is thickened.

4. Spread beef in prepared pie pan.

5. In a large bowl, combine eggs, cream, garlic, salt and pepper. Pour over beef.

6. Sprinkle with shredded cheese and bake 30 minutes, or until centre is set and cheese is browned.

7. Remove and let sit 5 minutes before slicing and serving.

8. Top with sour cream, chopped tomatoes and chopped avocado, if desired.

Nutrition Facts

Amount Per Serving (1 slice (1/8th of pie))

Calories 370Calories from Fat 250

% Daily Value*

Total Fat 27.8g43%

Total Carbohydrates 2.14g1%

Dietary Fiber 0.19g1%

Protein 24.1g48%

KETO SHEET PAN SALMON

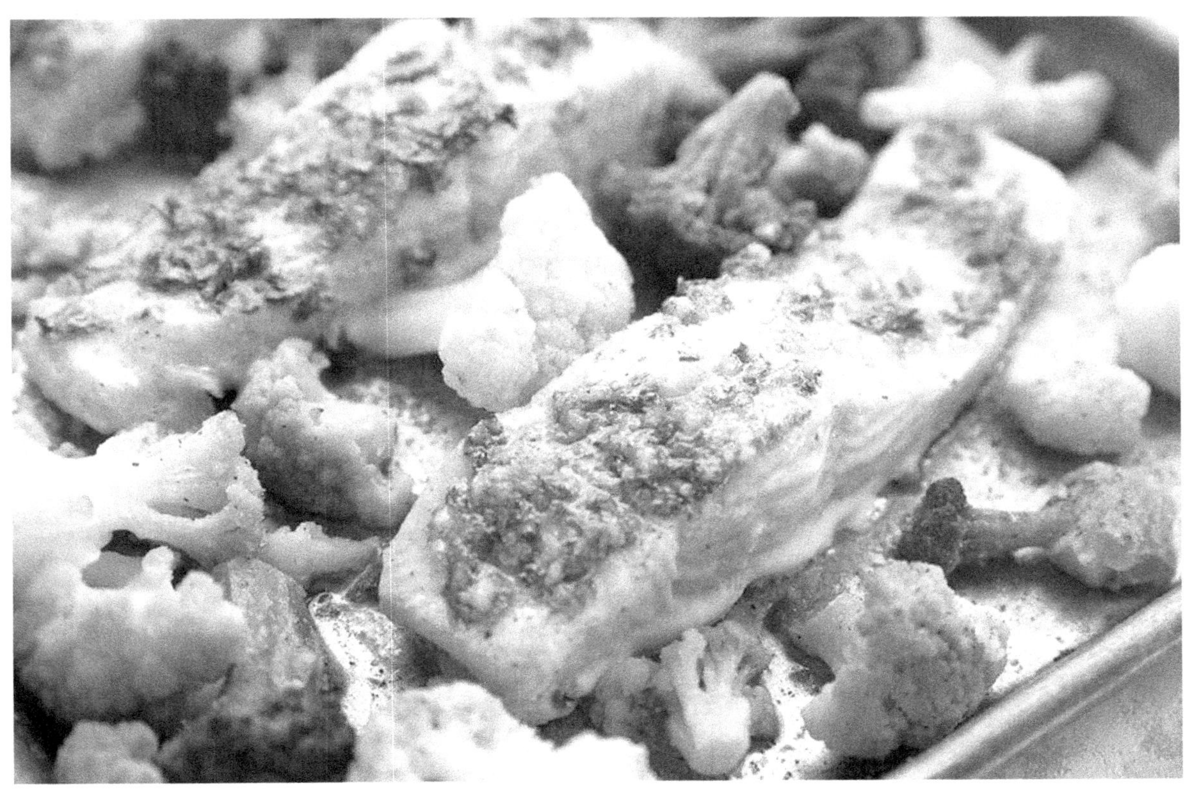

Easy Garlic Butter Salmon perfectly cooked keto salmon with a delicious drizzle of garlic herb butter. This single sheet pan meal takes only a few minutes of prep time and comes together in less than 30 minutes, start to finish.

It's the perfect low carb dinner for those hectic weeknights

Prep Time: 5 mins

Cook Time:22 mins

Total Time: 27 mins

Perfectly cooked salmon with a delicious drizzle of garlic herb butter.

A single sheet pan meal that comes together in less than 30 minutes, start to finish.

Servings: 4 servings

Calories: 450 kcal

Ingredients

- 1/4 cup butter divided
- 3 cloves garlic minced
- 2 tbsp chopped fresh parsley
- 1 lb cauliflower florets
- Salt and pepper

- 1 1/2 lb salmon filet cut into 4 equal portions

- 1 tsp grated lemon zest

- Lemon wedges for serving

Instructions

1. Preheat the oven to 400F and place 2 tbsp of the butter on a rimmed baking sheet. Place the baking sheet in the oven as it preheats.

2. Melt the remaining butter in a small bowl and whisk in the garlic, parsley and lemon zest.

3. Remove the pan from the oven when the butter is melted and add the cauliflower florets. Sprinkle with salt and pepper and toss to coat in the butter. Bake 10 minutes.

4. Remove the pan from the oven and make space for the salmon filets. Sprinkle with salt and pepper, then drizzle with plenty of the garlic butter.

5. Bake another 10 to 12 minutes, until the fish is opaque and flakes easily with a fork. How long will depend on how thick your filets are.

6. Serve hot with wedges of lemon.

Nutrition Facts

Amount Per Serving (1 serving = 1 piece of fish and some 1/4 of the cauliflower)

Calories 450Calories from Fat 214

% Daily Value*

Total Fat 23.8g37%

Total Carbohydrates 6.3g2%

Dietary Fiber 2.4g10%

Protein 36.9g74%

KETO SOUPS AND STEWS

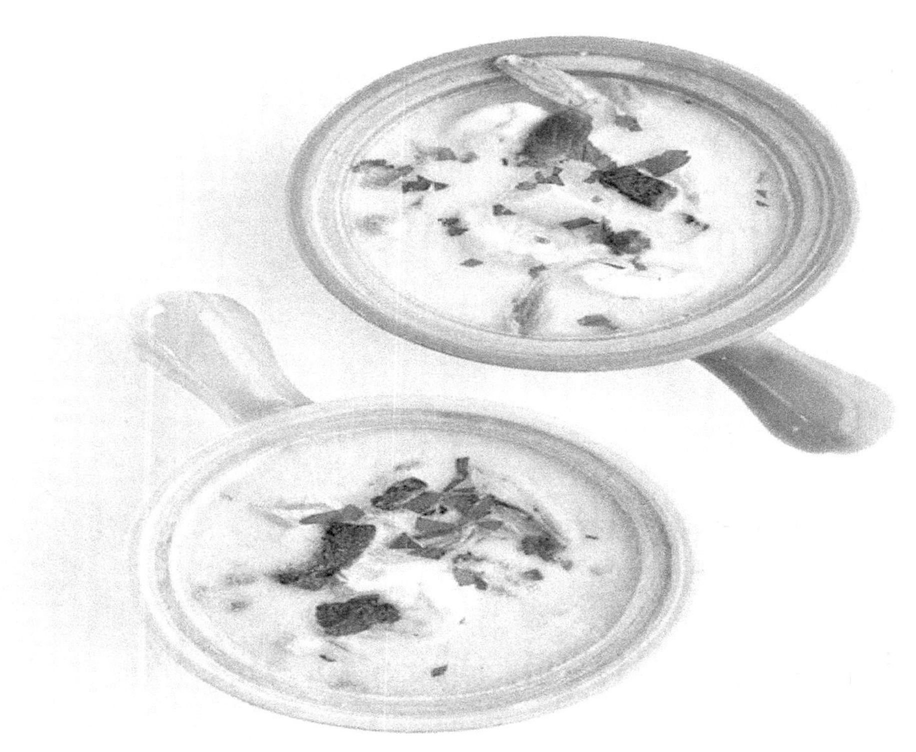

Shrimp and bacon come together in a creamy, rich soup that only takes a few minutes to make. It's weeknight comfort food! Keto recipe

Prep Time: 5 mins

Cook Time:25 mins

Total Time: 30 mins

Servings: 6 servings

Calories: 391 kcal

Ingredients

- 6 slices bacon chopped

- 1 medium turnip cut into ½-inch cubes

- ½ cup chopped onion

- 2 cloves garlic minced

- 2 cups chicken broth

- 1 cup heavy whipping cream

- 1 pound shrimp peeled and deveined, tails on or off

- ½ teaspoon Cajun seasoning

- Salt and pepper

- Chopped parsley for garnish

Instructions

1. In a large pot or Dutch oven over medium heat, cook the bacon until crisp. Using a slotted spoon, transfer to a paper towel-lined plate to drain, reserving the bacon fat in the pan.

2. Add the turnip and onion to the pan and saute until the onion is tender, about 5 minutes. Stir in the garlic and cook until fragrant, another minute or so. Pour in the chicken broth and simmer until the turnip is tender, about 10 minutes.

3. Stir in the cream and the shrimp and simmer until the shrimp is pink and cooked through, another 3 minutes or so. Add the Cajun seasoning and season to taste with salt and pepper.

4. Garnish with the bacon and chopped parsley upon serving.

Recipe Notes

Tip: Some Cajun seasoning has a lot of added salt. Be sure to taste your soup after adding the seasoning, before you add any additional salt and pepper.

Also make sure your seasoning has no added sugar or other fillers. We really like Slap Ya Mama seasoning blend. Yes, that's really what it's called!

Nutrition Facts

Amount Per Serving (1 serving = about 3/4 cup)

Calories 391Calories from Fat 287

% Daily Value*

Total Fat 31.9g49%

Total Carbohydrates 5.6g2%

Dietary Fiber 0.6g2%

Protein 16.5g33%

LOW CARB CHICKEN QUESADILLAS

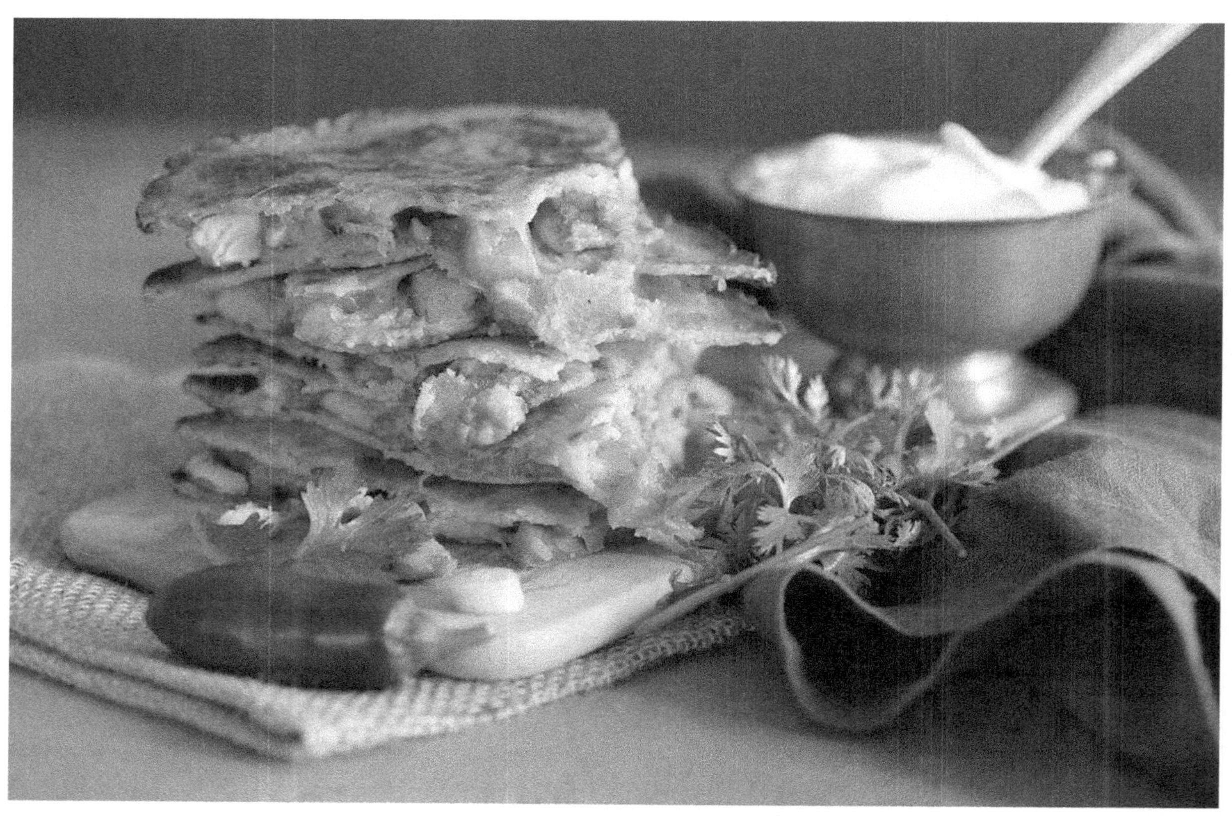

Prep Time: 15 mins

Cook Time: 20 mins

Total Time: 35 mins

This keto-friendly chicken quesadilla recipe is going to make you dance with joy. A grain-free low carb quesadilla that will surely satisfy that Mexican food craving.

Servings: 4 servings

Calories: 406 kcal

Ingredients

- 2 tbsp avocado oil divided

- 2 boneless skinless chicken thighs chopped into 1/2 inch pieces

- 1 tbsp taco seasoning

- 1/2 medium green pepper chopped into 1/2 inch pieces

- 2 medium green onions, thinly sliced white and light green parts only

- Salt and pepper to taste

- 2 packs KBosh Pizza Crusts

- 1 1/2 cups shredded cheddar or Mexican cheese

Instructions

1. In a large skillet over medium heat, heat 1 tablespoon of the avocado oil until shimmering but not smoking. Add the chicken and saute until mostly cooked through, about 5 minutes. Sprinkle with the taco seasoning.

2. Stir in the pepper and onions and continue to cook until the veggies are tender, another 3 to 5 minutes.

3. Transfer the chicken mixture to a bowl and wipe out the pan with a paper towel. Add another 1/2 tablespoons of the oil and reduce the heat to medium low.

4. Add one pizza crust to the pan and sprinkle with 1/2 cup of shredded cheese. Take half of the chicken filling and spread evenly over the cheese.

Sprinkle with another 1/4 cup of cheese and lay a second pizza crust on top.

5. Cover the pan and cook until the cheese is melted and the bottom is browned, 2 to 4 minutes. Carefully flip over and cook another 2 minutes. Remove and let cook a few minutes before cutting into slices.

6. Repeat with the remaining crusts, cheese, and filling.

Nutrition Facts

Low Carb Chicken Quesadillas

Amount Per Serving (1 serving = 1/2 of a quesadilla)

Calories 406Calories from Fat 230

% Daily Value*

Total Fat 25.6g39%

Total Carbohydrates 5.2g2%

Dietary Fiber 2.6g10%

Protein 28.6g57%

SAUSAGE ALFREDO WITH ZUCCHINI NOODLES

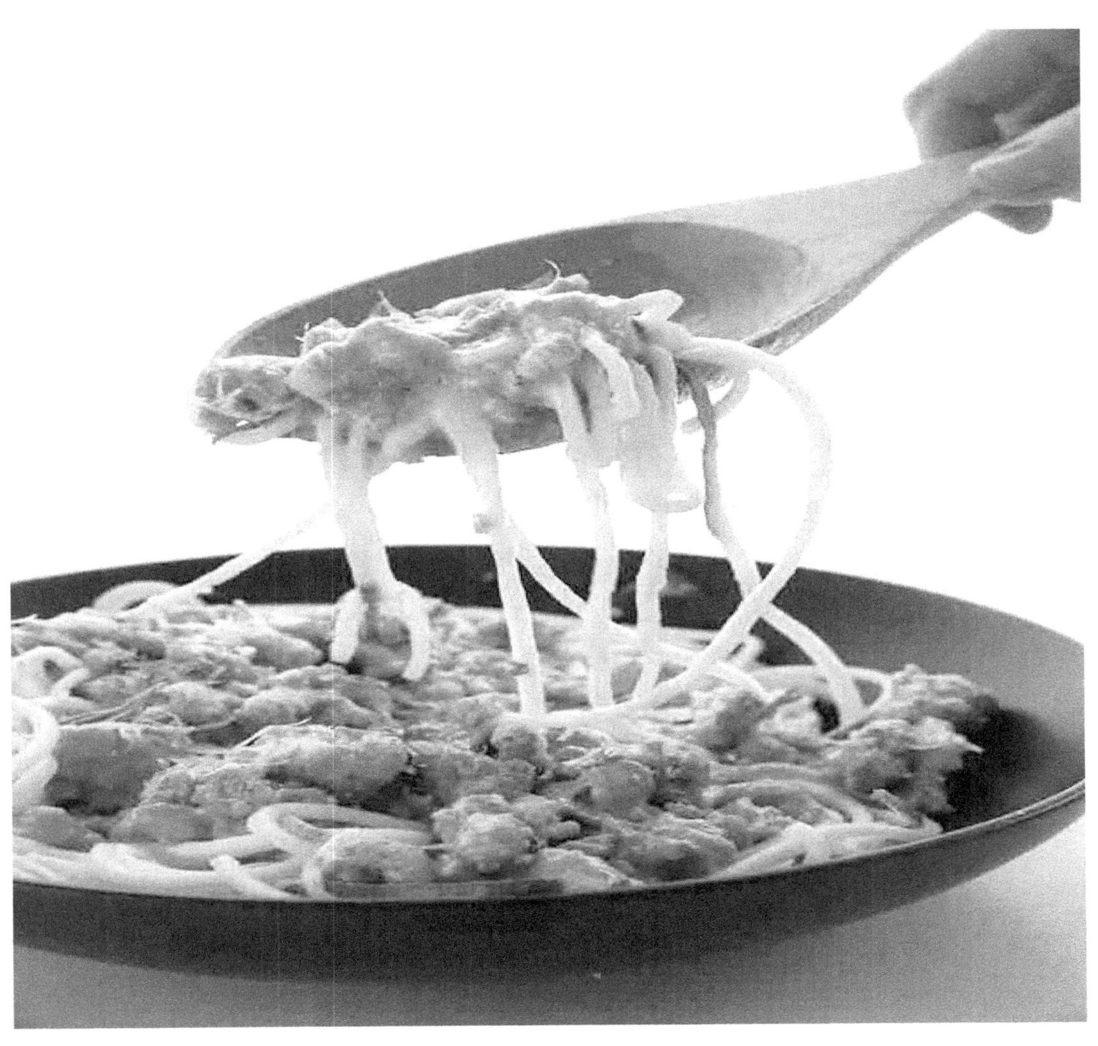

This keto alfredo sauce is creamy and rich, and perfect for serving over zoodles. With only 6 simple ingredients, it makes a satisfying low carb dinner the whole family will love.

Prep Time: 15 mins

Cook Time: 20 mins

Total Time: 31 mins

Servings: 4 servings

Calories: 583 kcal

Ingredients

- 12 ounces bulk hot Italian sausage

- 2 tbsp butter

- 3 cloves garlic minced

- 1 cup heavy whipping cream

- 1/2 cup freshly grated parmesan

- Salt and pepper

- 2 medium zucchini spiralized

Instructions

1. In a large skillet over medium heat, brown the sausage until cooked through, 5 to 8 minutes. Transfer to a bowl, leaving some of the grease in the pan.

2. Add the butter and let melt, then add the garlic. Saute until fragrant, about 1 minute. Add the cream and bring to a simmer. Reduce the heat and cook on low until thickened, 5 to 8 minutes, whisking frequently.

3. Whisk in the Parmesan and season with salt and pepper to taste. Add the sausage back in and whisk to combine. If your sauce ends up too thick as it cools, add a little extra cream if necessary.

4. Place the zucchini noodles in a large microwave-safe bowl and cook on high for 2 minutes, until just tender. Divide among 4 plates and top with sausage alfredo. Serve immediately.

Nutrition Facts

Amount Per Serving (1 serving = 1/4 of recipe)

Calories 583Calories from Fat 468

% Daily Value*

Total Fat 52g80%

Total Carbohydrates 6.1g2%

Dietary Fiber 1g4%

Protein 16g32%

LEMON DILL TUNA PATTIES

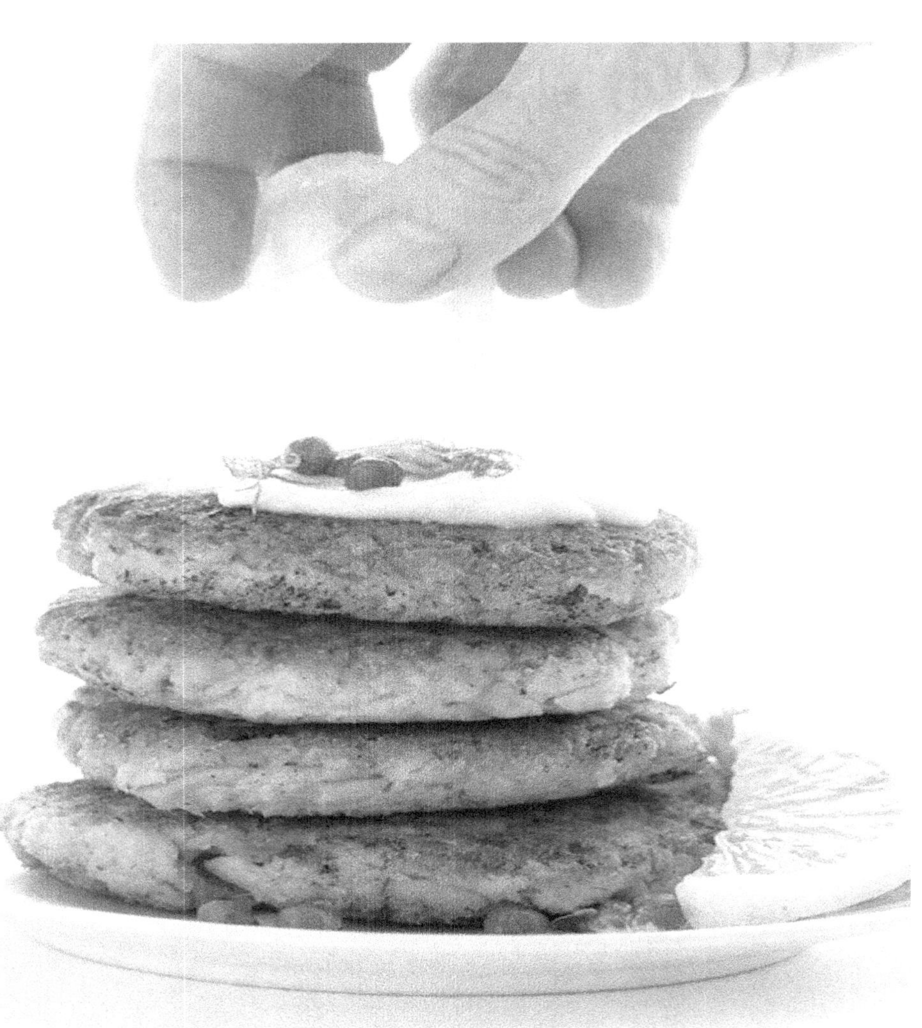

Prep Time: 10 mins

Cook Time: 10 mins

Total Time: 20 mins

I officially declare these the best tuna patties ever! These healthy keto tuna burgers are easy to make, delicious, and a very family friendly recipe. A great way to get a little more fish in your low carb diet. Less than 2g carbs per serving.

Servings: 8 patties

Calories: 215 kcal

Ingredients

- 4 5-ounce cans tuna drained

- 1/3 cup almond flour

- 2 medium green onions, chopped white and light green parts only

- 2 tbsp chopped fresh dill

- 1 tbsp lemon zest

- 3/4 tsp salt

- 1/2 tsp pepper

- 1/4 cup mayonnaise

- 1 large egg

- 1 tbsp freshly squeezed lemon juice

- 2 tbsp avocado oil

Instructions

1. In a large bowl, mix together all of the ingredients except the avocado oil until well combined. Form into 8 patties about 3/4 inch thick.

2. In a large skillet, heat 1 tbsp of the avocado oil over medium heat until shimmering. Add half of tuna patties and cook until golden brown on the bottom, about 3 to 4 minutes.

3. Carefully flip over and cook the other side another 3 to 4 minutes. Remove to a paper towel lined plate and repeat with the remaining oil and patties.

4. Top with mayo, lemon, and capers, if desired.

Nutrition Facts

Amount Per Serving (1 patty)

Calories 215Calories from Fat 128

% Daily Value*

Total Fat 14.2g22%

Total Carbohydrates 1.7g1%

Dietary Fiber 0.7g3%

Protein 22.2g44%

HOW TO MAKE KETO ASIAN STEAK BITES

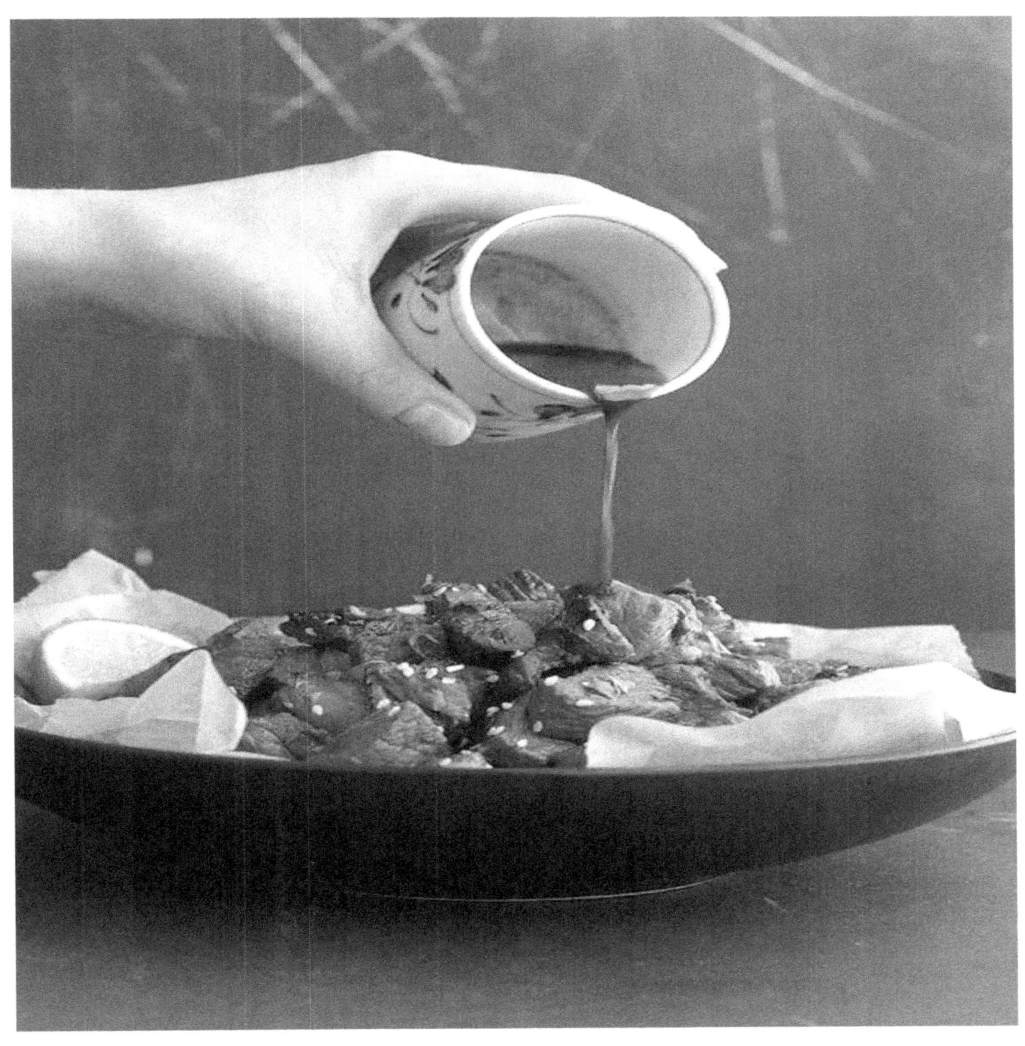

These Asian Steak Bites are tender, juicy, and oh so easy to make. A deceptively simple keto dinner recipe that the whole family loves. Paleo and dairy-free too!

Prep Time: 10 mins

Cook Time: 10 mins

Marinating Time: 30 mins

Total Time: 20 mins

Servings: 6 people

Calories: 280 kcal

Ingredients

- 1 1/2 lbs sirloin steak

- 1/4 cup coconut aminos or soy sauce

- 1 tbsp Swerve Sweetener

- 2 cloves garlic minced

- 1/2 tsp ground ginger

- 1/4 tsp red pepper flakes

- 2 tbsp sesame oil

- 2 tsp toasted sesame seeds

- chopped cilantro for garnish

Instructions

1. Cut the steak into small cubes no more than 1 inch in size. Try to do this as evenly as possible so the bites cook evenly. Set the steak bites in a medium bowl.

2. In a small bowl, whisk together the coconut aminos, sweetener, garlic, ginger, and red pepper flakes. Pour over the steak bites and toss to coat. Let marinate 30 minutes at room temperature or 2 hours in the fridge.

3. Heat a large skillet over medium high heat. Once hot, add 1 tablespoon of the sesame oil. Using a slotted spoon, add half of the steak bites in a single layer. Let them cook undisturbed for about 2 minutes, then quickly flip them over and cook on the second side for another minute or so. They should be seared on the outside but still a little pink and tender in the center.

4. Transfer to a bowl and repeat with the remaining oil and the remaining steak bites.

5. Once all the steak is cooked and removed from the pan, pour the reserved marinade into the pan and bring to a boil. Cook until reduced and thickened, 4 to 5 minutes. Pour over the steak bites or serve on the side.

6. Garnish with toasted sesame seeds and cilantro.

Recipe Notes

If you use coconut aminos, you may want to add a little salt to the finished recipe.

Nutrition Facts

Asian Steak Bites

Amount Per Serving (1 1/6th of recipe)

Calories 280Calories from Fat 152

% Daily Value*

Total Fat 16.9g26%

Total Carbohydrates 2.5g1%

Dietary Fiber 0.1g0%

Protein 23.1g46%

EASY CAPRESE CHICKEN

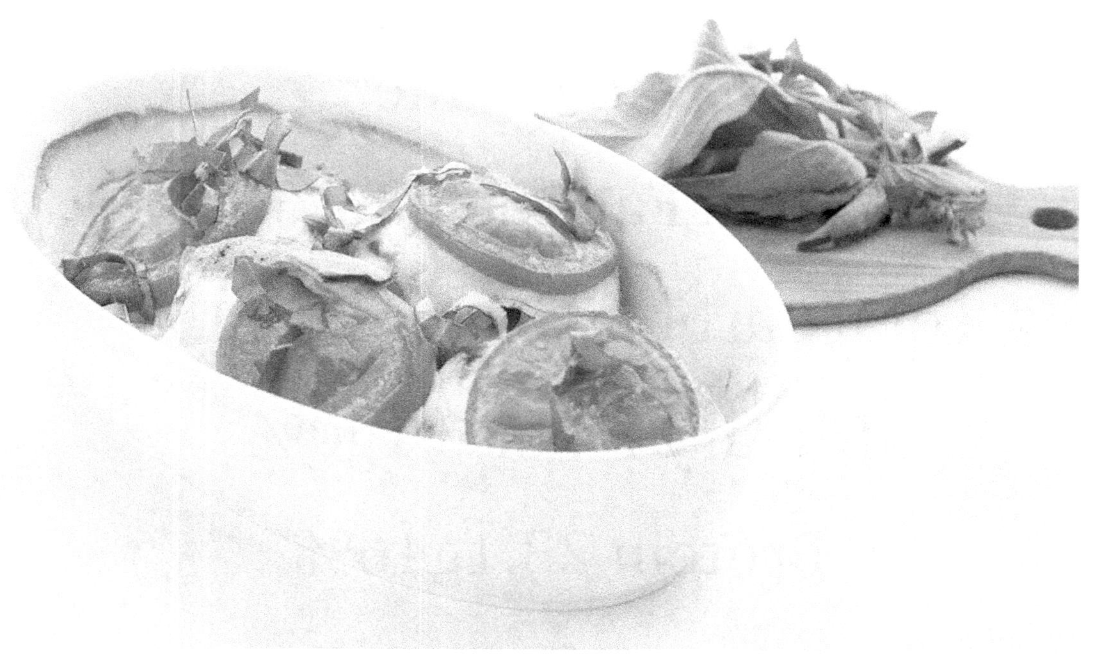

Prep Time: 5 mins

Cook Time: 35 mins

Total Time:40 mins

Trust me, this Easy Chicken Caprese is about to become your new favorite keto dinner recipe. Simple to make with 5 ingredients and the whole family loves it. It's a delicious way to use some of the fresh summer produce and has less than 2g total carbs per serving.

Servings: 4 servings

Calories: 315 kcal

Ingredients

- 2 tbsp avocado oil

- 5 boneless skinless chicken thighs

- Salt and pepper

- 6 ounces fresh mozzarella sliced into 5 or 6 slices

- 1 medium tomato sliced into 5 or 6 slices (as many as you have thighs)

- 1/4 cup fresh basil chopped

Instructions

1. Preheat oven to 375F.

2. In a large skillet, heat the oil until over medium heat until shimmering. Sprinkle chicken thighs with salt and pepper and add in a single layer to pan. Sear on the first side until golden brown, about 2 to 3 minutes, then sear on the second side another 2 to 3 minutes.

3. Arrange chicken in a single layer in a medium casserole dish or glass baking pan. Top each chicken thigh with a slice of fresh mozzarella, then top each with a slice of tomato.

4. Bake 25 to 28 minutes, until cheese is melted and bubbling and chicken is cooked through. Turn on broiler for 2 or 3 minutes to brown the top of the cheese.

5. Remove from oven and sprinkle with fresh basil.

Nutrition Facts

Amount Per Serving (1 thigh)

Calories 315Calories from Fat 168

% Daily Value*

Total Fat 18.7g29%

Total Carbohydrates 1.63g1%

Dietary Fiber 0.4g2%

Protein 35.7g71%

INSTANT POT SALSA CHICKEN

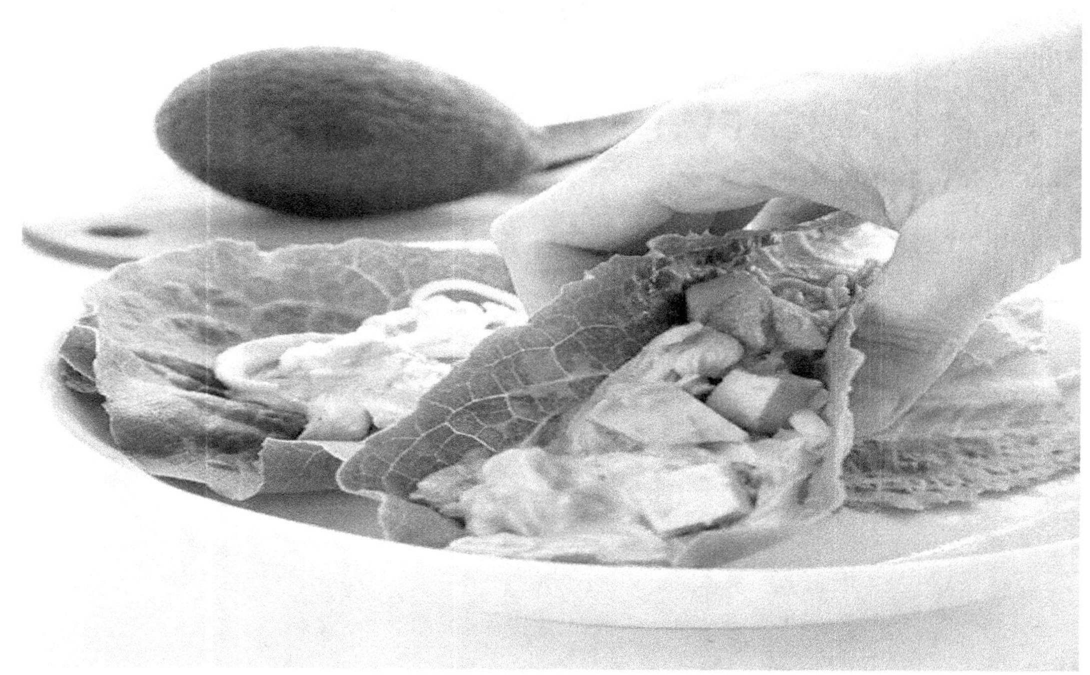

This is what I like to call a dump-and-run recipe. It really is one of those insanely easy Instant Pot recipes where you can dump everything in, turn the machine on, and walk away. The prep time is so minimal as to be non-existent. But a few notes to make it truly low carb and healthy.

Prep Time: 5 mins

Cook Time: 30 mins

Total Time: 35 mins

This creamy Instant Pot salsa chicken is officially my kids' new favorite keto dinner. 5 simple ingredients and it's so easy to make, it will quickly become your favorite low carb dinner recipe too!

Servings: 6 servings

Calories: 244 kcal

Ingredients

- 2 lbs boneless skinless chicken thighs
- 3 tbsp taco seasoning
- Salt and pepper

- 4 ounces cream cheese cut into chunks

- 1 cup salsa mild or hot, your preference

- 1/4 cup chicken broth

Instructions

1. Place the chicken thighs in the bottom of the Instant Pot. Sprinkle with taco seasoning and a little additional salt and pepper.

2. Add the cream cheese, salsa, and broth and lock the lid into place. Use the manual setting and set the Instant Pot on high for 20 minutes. Once it's finished cooking, allow the pressure to release naturally for 15 minutes.

3. Use the vent to release any remaining pressure and then remove the lid. Remove the chicken to a plate and use an immersion blender to puree the sauce until smooth. Alternatively, you can transfer the sauce to a regular blender and puree.

4. Shred the chicken with two forks and add back into the pot. Toss to coat in the creamy sauce. Serve with lettuce wraps and top with chopped avocados and shredded cheddar cheese.

Recipe Notes

You can make this easily in a crockpot too. 3 to 4 hours on low will do, unless you are doubling the recipe.

Nutrition Facts

Keto Salsa Chicken Recipe

Amount Per Serving

Calories 244Calories from Fat 89

% Daily Value*

Total Fat 9.9g15%

Total Carbohydrates 4.2g1%

Dietary Fiber 1.6g6%

Protein 30.2g60%

EASY GREEK SHRIMP

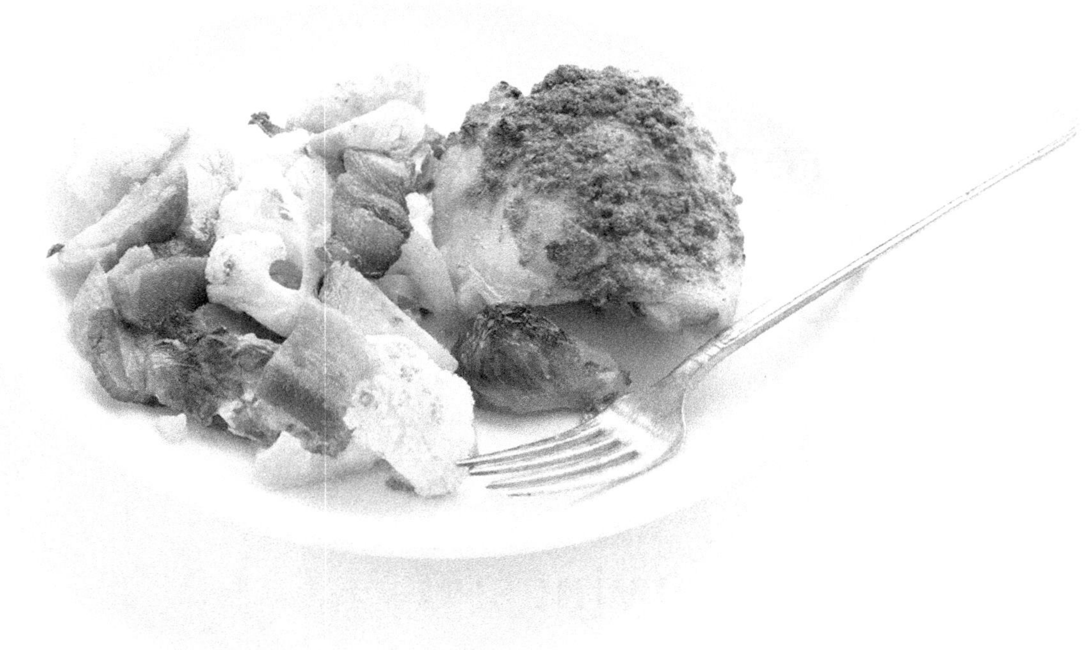

This light and easy low carb Greek Shrimp recipe is a wonderful summer meal. Enjoy it al fresco with your friends and family

Prep Time: 10 mins

Cook Time: 25 mins

Total Time: 35 mins

Servings: 6

Calories: 175 kcal

Ingredients

- 2 tbsp avocado oil

- 2 cloves garlic minced

- 1 15- ounce can diced tomatoes drained

- 1 tsp salt

- 3/4 tsp black pepper

- 1/2 tsp red pepper flakes

- 1 1/2 lbs medium shrimp peeled and deveined

- 1/2 cup freshly grated parmesan

- 3/4 cup crumbled feta cheese divided

- Fresh parsley for garnish

Instructions

1. Preheat the oven to 375F.

2. In a large oven-proof saute pan, heat the oil over medium heat until shimmering. Add the garlic and sauté 30 seconds. Stir in the tomatoes, salt, pepper and red pepper flakes and bring to a simmer. Cook 5 minutes.

3. Lay the shrimp in a single layer over the tomatoes and sprinkle with the parmesan and 1/2 cup of the feta. Place the pan in the oven and bake until the shrimp is pink and cooked through, 10 to 15 minutes.

4. Remove and sprinkle with the remaining feta and some fresh chopped parsley. Serve over cauliflower rice.

Nutrition Facts

Easy Greek Shrimp

Amount Per Serving

Calories 175Calories from Fat 90

% Daily Value*

Total Fat 9.96g15%

Total Carbohydrates 5.19g2%

Dietary Fiber 0.96g4%

Protein 19.67g39%

EASY PIZZA CHICKEN

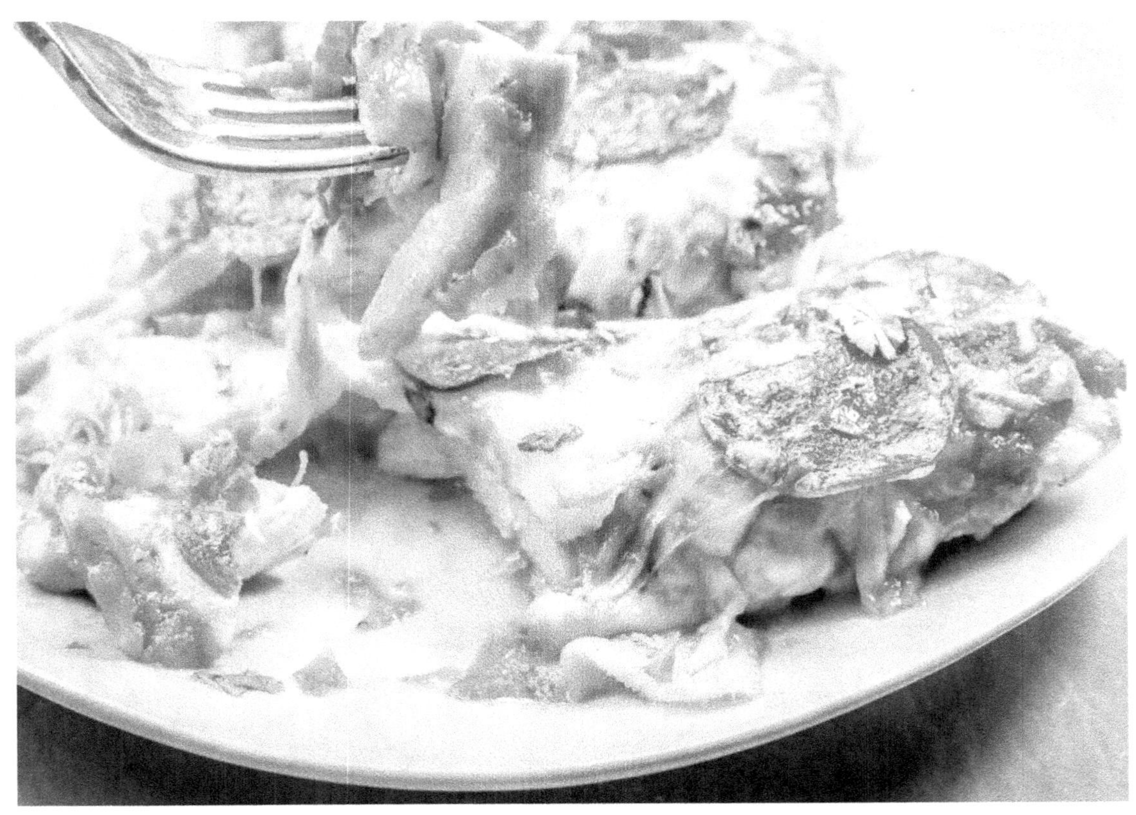

That's really it. You can't beat the convenience and flavor of this keto pizza chicken recipe. Hope your family loves it as much as mine does!

Juicy low carb chicken thighs smothered in pizza sauce, pepperoni, and mozzarella. This easy one-pan meal will be a hit with your whole family.

Prep Time: 5 mins

Cook Time: 30 mins

Total Time: 35 mins

Servings: 6 servings

Calories: 443 kcal

Ingredients

- 2 tbsp avocado or olive oil

- 2 lb boneless skinless chicken thighs

- Salt and pepper

- 1 cup pizza sauce or marinara sauce (make sure it has no added sugar)

- 2 ounces sliced pepperoni (I like this one from Applegate)

- 1 1/2 to 2 cups shredded mozzarella

Instructions

1. Preheat oven to 350F.

2. Heat oil in a large 12-inch skillet over medium heat (if it's a cast-iron skillet, be generous with your oil to avoid sticking). Sprinkle chicken thighs with salt and pepper and to pan. Cook until lightly browned, 2 to 4 minutes per side.

3. Pour pizza sauce over chicken thighs, spreading to coat. Arrange pepperoni over chicken and sprinkle with mozzarella.

4. Bake 25 minutes, then turn on broiler for a minute or two until cheese is bubbly and browned in spots.

Nutrition Facts

Calories 443Calories from Fat 242

% Daily Value*

Total Fat 26.84g41%

Cholesterol 202mg67%

Total Carbohydrates 3.59g1%

Dietary Fiber 0.61g2%

Protein 35.7g71%

ALMOND BUTTER KRUNCH KETO CEREAL RECIPE

Ingredients

- 1 egg

- 3/4 cup almond butter

- 1/2 cup of your favorite keto friendly sweetener. I prefer Lakanto Monkfruit for this recipe but I've also tried Pyure All purpose blend Erythritol, and Xylitol too

Instructions

1. Almond Butter Krunch Keto Cereal Recipe Instructions

2. Preheat the oven to 350 degrees.

3. In a medium size bowl, add all the ingredients in a bowl and mix them all together until it's well combined.

4. Using a spatula, press the dough into the silicone gummy bear molds as seen in the video below.

5. Place the filled silicone molds on a cookie sheet. The molds are flimsy and this will help carry them in and out of the oven.

6. You will bake these cookies for about 12 to 15 minutes or until golden brown.

7. Allow them to cool down for about 5 minutes before removing them from the silicone molds.

8. Store them in an airtight container in the fridge if you have any left over.

9. We tend to split this recipe into 4 to 6 servings.

KETO MAPLE FRENCH TOAST BAGELS RECIPE

The excitement of breakfast time just got even better with these Keto Maple French Toast Bagels! A wonderful cross between a classic french toast plate and a yummy warm bread bagel.

Prep Time:10 minutes

Cook Time:20 minutes

Servings: 12 servings

Calories: 164kcal

Ingredients

- 6 tbs Bacon Grease

- 6 tbs Coconut Flour By Bob's Red Mill

- 6 tbs Psyllium Husk Powder By Healthworks

- 6 tbs Powdered Monkfruit Sweetener By Lakanto

- 1 tbs Baking Powder

- 1 tsp Fine Pink Salt

- 6 Large Eggs whisked

- 12 tbs Maple Flavored Syrup By Lakanto

Instructions

1. Preheat oven to 350 degrees.

2. In a large mixing bowl- Add melted/warm grease.

3. Add all dry ingredients, mixing well to break up any clumps.

4. Then add in the eggs and Lakanto Maple Syrup, mix until well incorporated.

5. Fill 2 6-ring donut pans with batter.

6. Smooth out and tap on counter to release any trapped air bubbles.

7. Bake on middle rack for 18-20 minutes.

8. Remove from the oven and let cool completely before popping out.

9. Store bagels in the fridge or freezer for later!

Notes

If you don't have bacon grease, you could use butter or oil- but I really enjoy the flavor it gives from the bacon grease.

Enjoy them with cream cheese, peanut butter, SF maple syrup or jam. Any way you like them, breakfast is going to be delicious!

I tried alternatively baking them in a muffin top pan, and they were just like a pancake. I imagine a mini bread loaf pan would do just as well.

Nutrition

Serving: 1g | Calories: 164kcal | Carbohydrates: 16g | Protein: 4g | Fat: 9g | Fiber: 10g

INSTANT POT PULLED PORK

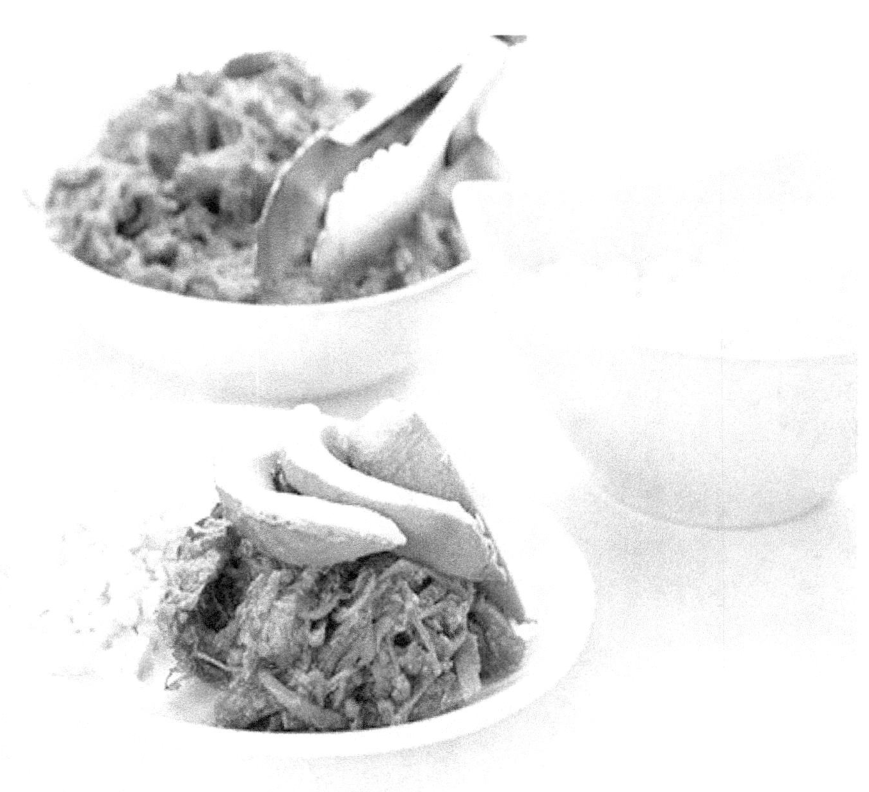

Prep Time: 15 mins

Cook Time: 1 hr 5 mins

Total Time: 1 hr 20 mins

This Instant Pot Pulled Pork Recipe is going to become your favorite new keto dinner! So easy and simple to make, with a sugar free BBQ Sauce for extra flavor. Paleo and dairy-free, and only 2g total carbs per serving.

Servings: 10 servings

Calories: 397 kcal

Ingredients

3 to 4 lb pork butt

Salt and pepper

2 tbsp bacon grease (or any oil/butter you prefer)

1 tbsp chile powder

1 tsp ground cumin

1 tsp garlic powder

3/4 cup chicken broth

1 recipe Easy Sugar Free BBQ Sauce

Instructions

Pat the pork roast dry with a clean rag, then chop into large chunks for faster cooking. Sprinkle generously all over with salt and pepper.

Turn the instant pot on to the saute function and add the bacon grease. Once melted and hot, add half the pork chunks and brown on all sides. Remove from the pan and repeat with the remaining chunks.

Place all the pork back in the pot and sprinkle with the chili powder, cumin, and garlic. Pour in the chicken broth and seal the lid. Make sure the vent is on seal.

Set the Instant Pot to manual high for 45 minutes. Once cooking is complete, let the pressure release naturally for another 15 to 20 minutes.

Transfer the pork to a large bowl and shred with two forks.

Add the BBQ sauce and toss to combine.

Season with additional salt and pepper

to taste.

Recipe Notes

To make in the oven: Preheat the oven to

300F. Heat the bacon grease in a large

Dutch oven over medium heat and

brown the pork chunks. Add in the

spices and chicken broth (add more

chicken broth for the oven method.

About 1 1/4 cups will do).

Cover and transfer to the oven and let cook 3 hours. Then remove and shred the pork and toss with the BBQ sauce.

Nutrition Facts

Instant Pot Pulled Pork

Amount Per Serving   (1 serving = 1/10th of recipe)

Calories 397 Calories from Fat 228

% Daily Value*

Total Fat 25.3g 39%

Total Carbohydrates 2.1g 1%

Dietary Fiber 0.6g 2%

Protein 34.7g 69%

INCONCLUSION

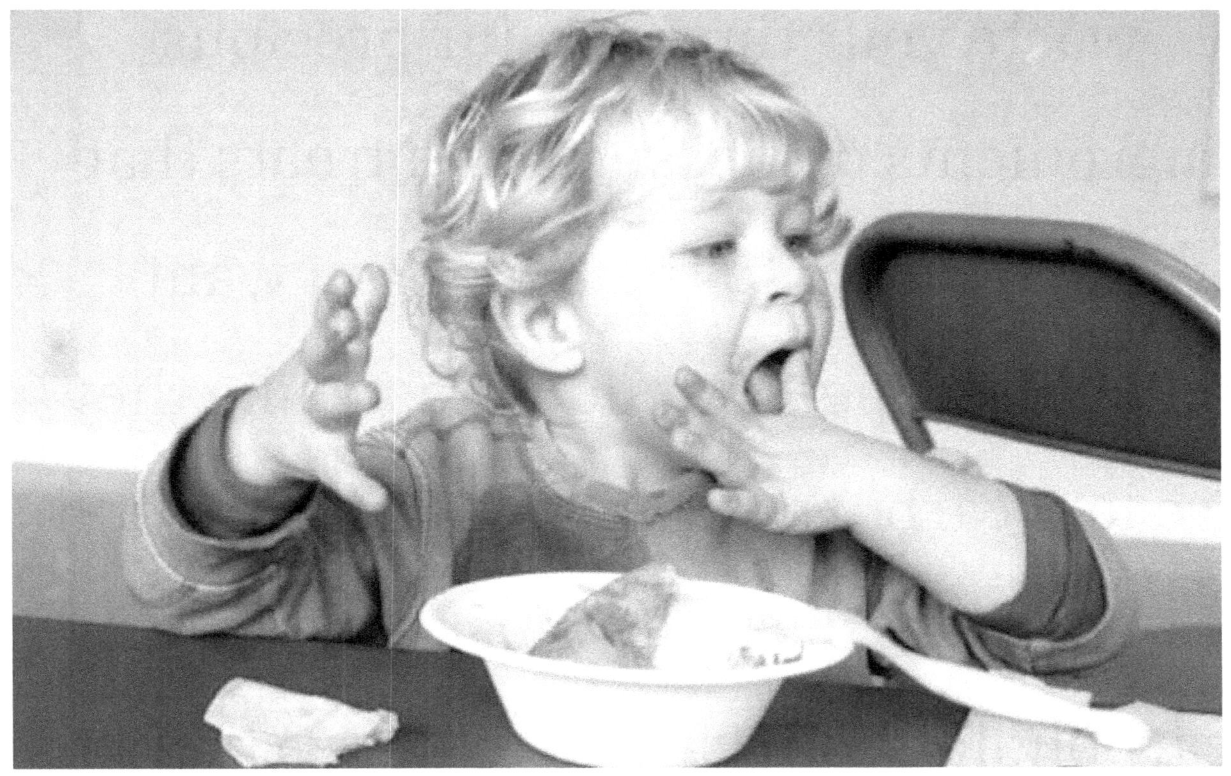

Let's be honest not all keto recipes are created equal and you don't want to waste your time or your precious ingredients on desserts and treats that don't live up to the hype. You want reliable recipes that don't taste like they are low carb. You want desserts that will impress even the most diehard carboholic. You want keto desserts that no one will know are good for them. Unless you choose to tell them. And that, my friend, is up to you. It can be our little secret.

As a passionate baker who made it my mission in life to make EASY FRIENDLY RECIPES that taste just as good, or better, than the real thing. But over the past few years, I've cut back my carbs more and more and fully embraced the ketogenic lifestyle.

THANKS FOR YOU

NANCY KAYLI